A PATIENT'S GUIDE TO UNDERSTANDING ADVANCED HEALTH CARE DIRECTIVES

I0410057

By Maureen Kroning MSN RN

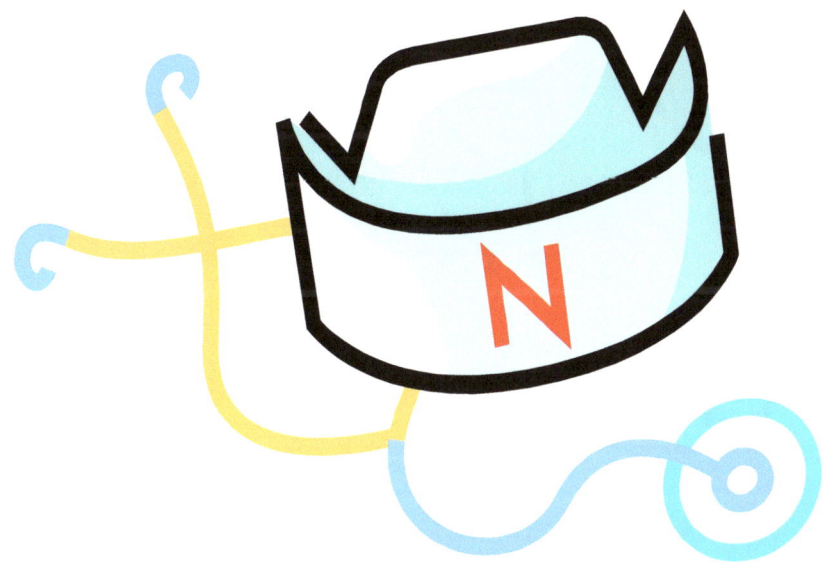

Dedication

This handbook is dedicated to patients, families, communities and the nurses that touch their lives each and every day.

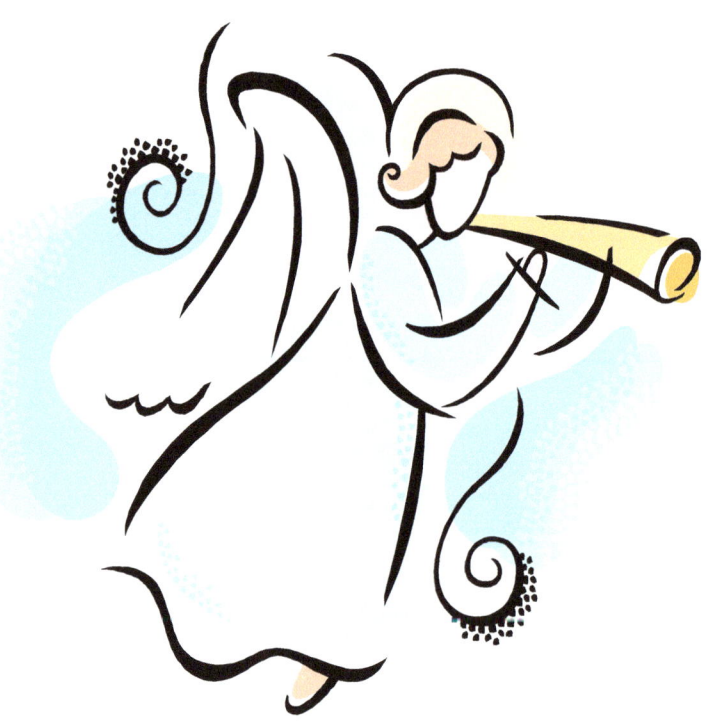

What are Advanced Health Care Directives (AHCD)?

- AHCD are legal documents that communicate to your healthcare provider(s) the medical care you wish to receive in the event you are no longer able due to illness or you are incapacitated.

- It is important that you tell your doctor and nurse your healthcare wishes.

- You may also choose to tell your family and friends your healthcare wishes.

What is included in AHCD?

- A Living Will

- A living will can include: A Do not Resuscitate (DNR) order or even a Do Not Intubate (DNI) order.

- A Healthcare Power of Attorney

- A Healthcare Power of Attorney can also be known as: a health care proxy, a surrogate, representative or a durable healthcare power of attorney.

A Living Will

- A Living Will is a legal document that communicates to your healthcare provider what medical care you want or do not want in the event that you are too ill or incapacitated.

- This document gives you the right to accept or refuse medical care.

Healthcare Power of Attorney

- A Healthcare Power of Attorney is a document that allows you to give the name of someone you trust to make health care decisions for you in the event you are no longer able to.

- This person or agent can make decisions for you only after your doctor has determined that you are unable to do so yourself.

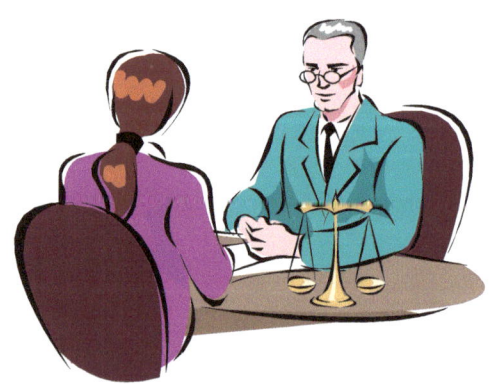

Do Not Resuscitate (DNR)

- A DNR is a legal order that tells your healthcare provider that you do not wish to have Cardio Pulmonary Resuscitation (CPR) if your heart stops beating or you stop breathing.

- It is important to tell your doctor or nurse if you have a DNR order.

- You may decide at any time to add a DNR order to your living will.

Do not Resuscitate (DNR)

- It is important to understand that having a DNR order does not mean that you will not receive medical treatment while in the hospital.

- You can determine what types of treatments you want or do not want.

- Please remember to be as specific as possible by putting your wishes in writing to avoid any confusion.

What could a DNR mean?

- If you stop breathing (respiratory arrest) or your heart stops (cardiac arrest) you will not receive: chest compressions, respirations, intubation, ventilation, defibrillation, or resuscitation medications. However, you should be specific to what you want or do not want.

- If your heart does not stop or you do not go into respiratory arrest you will still be treated for any injuries, pain and difficulty with breathing, bleeding and other medical conditions.

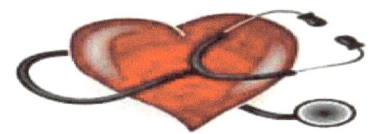

Do Not Intubate (DNI)

- You may decide you want CPR but do not want to have an endotracheal tube inserted. This is what a DNI means.

- A DNI has to be clearly stated in your living will.

- A DNI must be put in writing so that your doctor and nurse can follow your wishes.

Medical Treatments to Consider

- Cardio Pulmonary Resuscitation (CPR)
- Endotracheal/tracheal Intubation
- Ventilator
- Oxygen Therapy
- Dialysis
- Tube Feedings
- Donation of Organs and/or Tissues

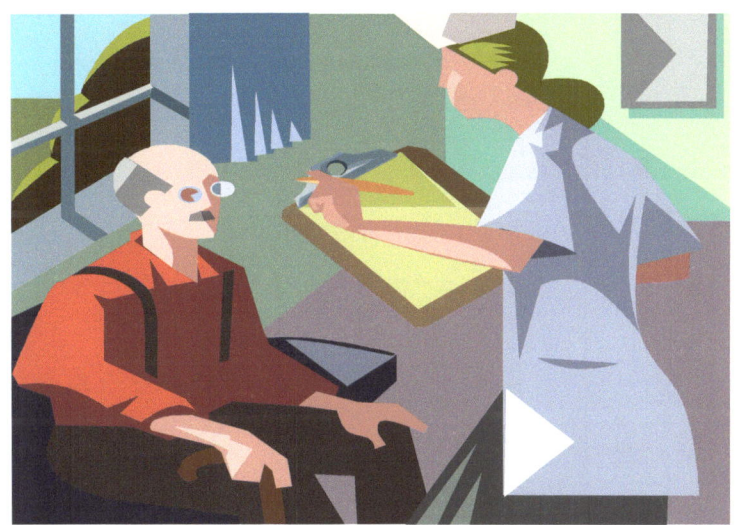

Cardio Pulmonary Resuscitation (CPR)

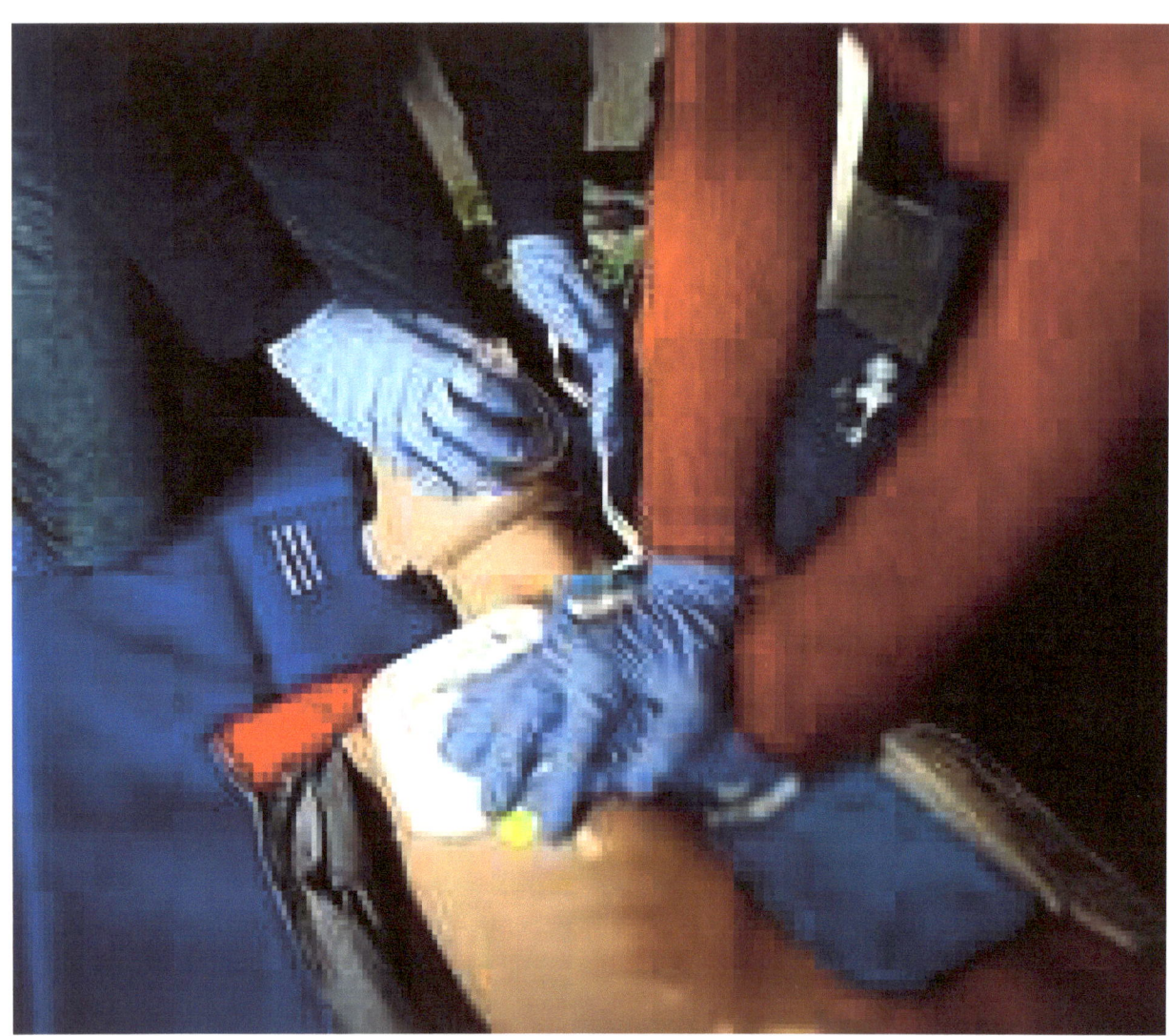

Cardio Pulmonary Resuscitation (CPR)

- Is an emergency procedure.

- The chest is compressed manually.

- The compressions send oxygenated blood to the heart and brain.

- Assisted breaths may also be done to put air into the lungs.

- CPR helps prevent cell death and brain damage.

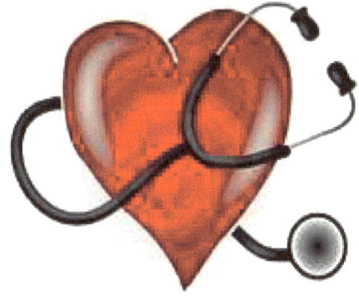

How effective is CPR?

- Studies show variation in CPR effectiveness depending on whom and where it is performed as well as the age of the patient.

- Studies show CPR alone results in few complete recoveries and serious complications may develop as a result.

- If your heart stops, CPR should be started as soon as possible. If you do not wish to have CPR make sure you have this in writing.

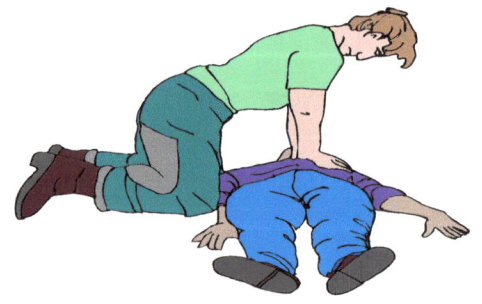

Endotracheal Tube

- Placement of an endotracheal tube is called intubation.

- A flexible plastic tube is inserted into your trachea through the mouth.

- This tube is placed into your trachea (windpipe) to keep your airway open.

- The endotracheal tube can be used to both administer oxygen and certain medications.

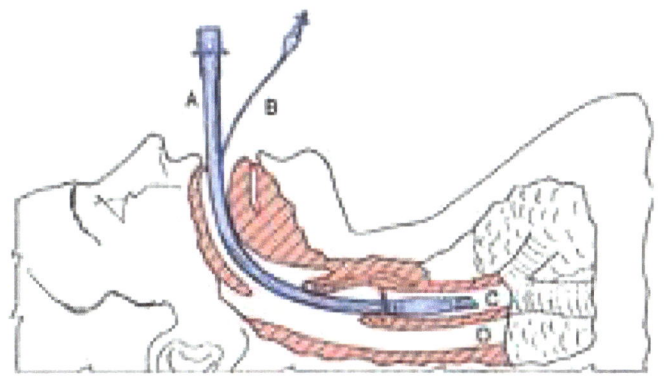

Endotracheal Tube

- The tube will be secured to the face and connected to an oxygen source, such as an ambo bag or a mechanical ventilator.

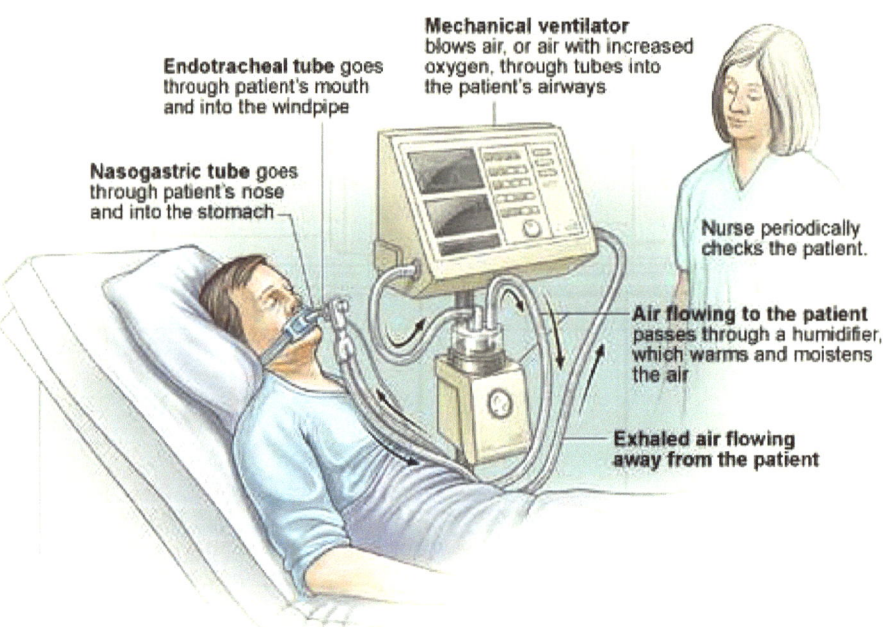

Mechanical ventilator blows air, or air with increased oxygen, through tubes into the patient's airways

Endotracheal tube goes through patient's mouth and into the windpipe

Nasogastric tube goes through patient's nose and into the stomach

Nurse periodically checks the patient.

Air flowing to the patient passes through a humidifier, which warms and moistens the air

Exhaled air flowing away from the patient

Complications associated with an endotracheal tube

- Complications can be minor, severe, long-lasting and even permanent.

- Some of the complications that can occur include: vocal cord damage, esophageal tear, nerve damage and fluid in the lungs.

A Ventilator

- A ventilator is a machine that attaches to the airway tube to move air into and out of the lungs if you are unable to breathe or breathing insufficiently. This is called mechanical ventilation.

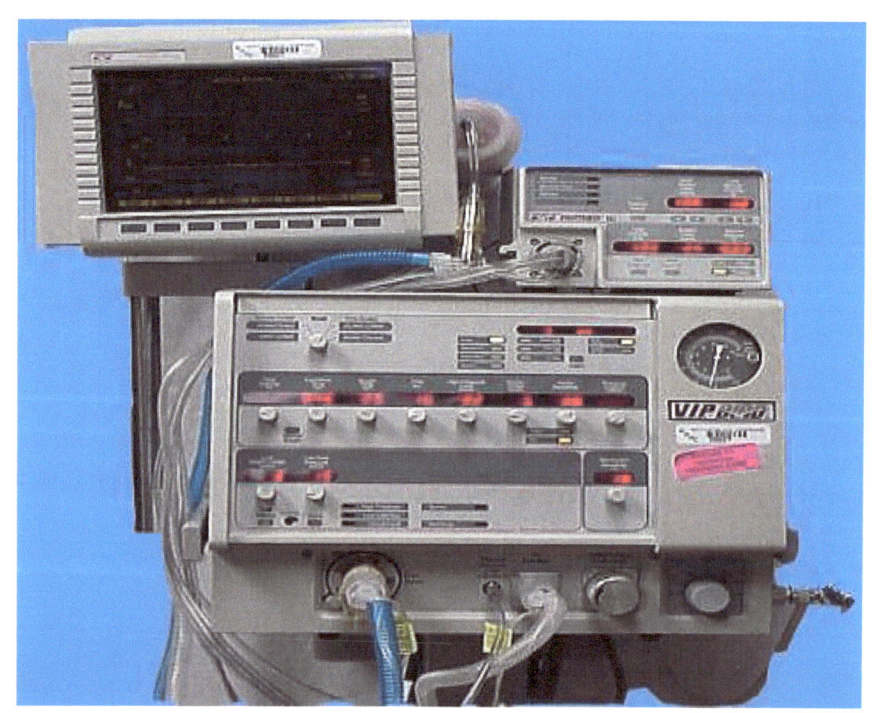

Complications of Mechanical Ventilator

- Pneumonia is both a common and serious complication.
- Sinus infection
- Air leaking into the space between the lungs and chest wall and air being pushed into the lungs with too much pressure can cause the lungs to collapse.
- High levels of oxygen can damage the lungs.
- Damage to the vocal cords as a result of the breathing tube.

Oxygen Therapy

Oxygen is needed for every cell in your body to function.

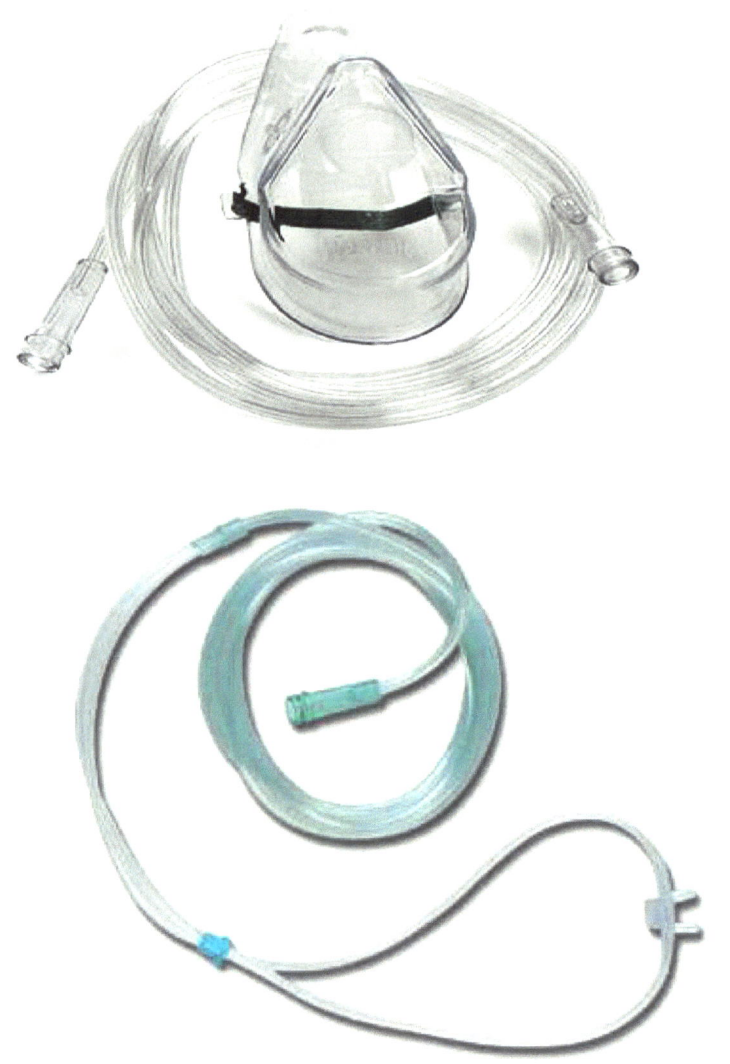

Complications of Oxygen Therapy

- Dry and/or bloody nose

- Skin irritation from the nasal cannula or face mask

- Fatigue (tiredness)

- Morning headaches

Dialysis

- A Dialysis machine takes away waste and excess water from the blood and is used when the kidneys fail to function properly.

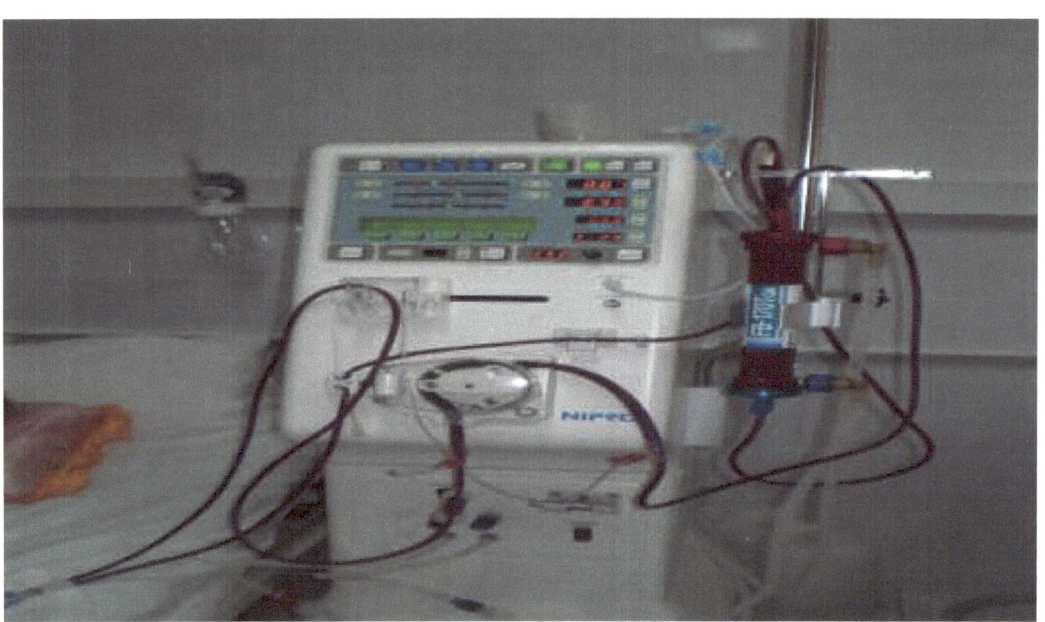

Complications of Dialysis

- Access complications

- Heart disease

- Vascular disease

- Fluid overload

- Malnutrition

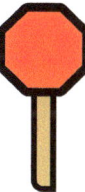

Enteral Tube Feedings

- Feedings administered into the intestine to ensure adequate nutrition.

- Administered through tubes such as: nasogastric, small-bore, gastrostomy or jejunostomy.

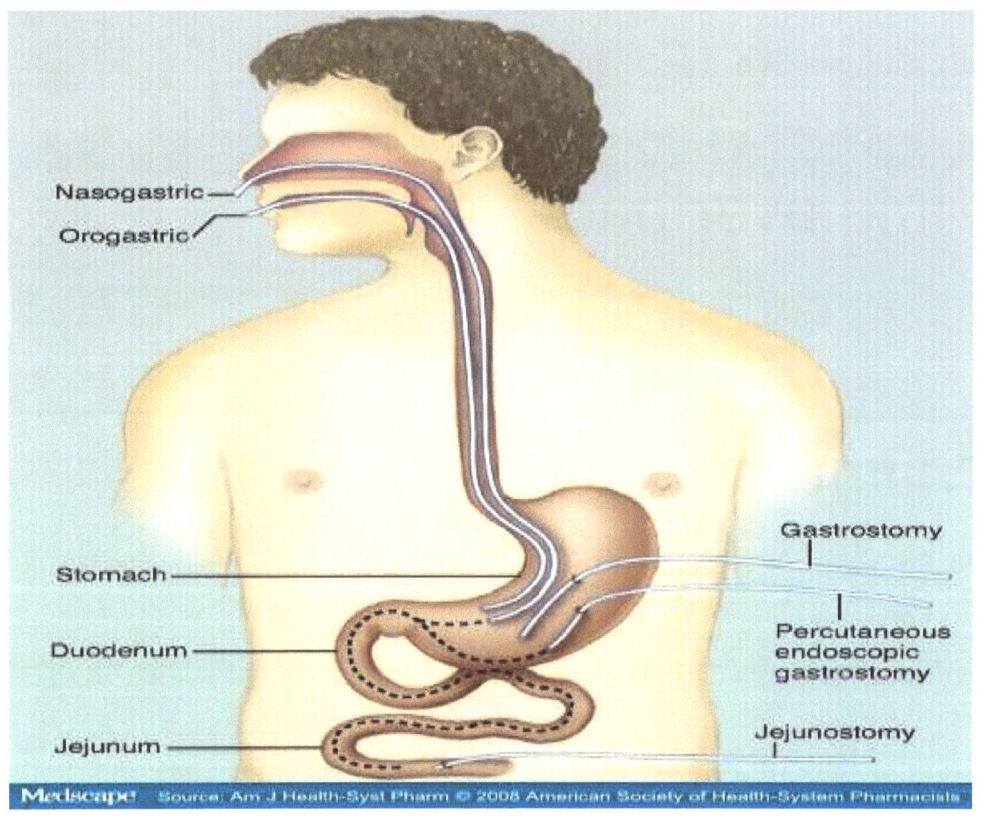

Nasogastric
Orogastric
Stomach
Duodenum
Jejunum
Gastrostomy
Percutaneous endoscopic gastrostomy
Jejunostomy

Medscape   Source: Am J Health-Syst Pharm © 2008 American Society of Health-System Pharmacists

Complications of Enteral Tube Feedings

- Gas, bloating, cramping
- Air in the tube
- Diarrhea
- Nausea, vomiting
- Constipation
- Aspiration
- Metabolic

Donation of Organs and/or Tissues

- Removal of healthy organs/ tissues from one person for transplantation into another.

- It is estimated that one donor can save or help up to 50 people.

- You can donate: kidneys, heart, liver, pancreas, intestines, lungs, skin, bone and bone marrow and cornea.

- Let your family/healthcare providers know your wishes.

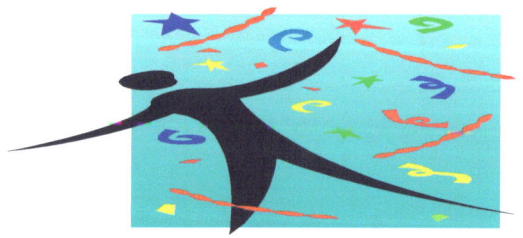

Five Wishes

- Five Wishes is a US National Advanced Directive that was created by an organization called Aging with Dignity.

- This directive considers not only your medical wishes but your spiritual needs as well.

- The first two wishes are part of your AHCD.

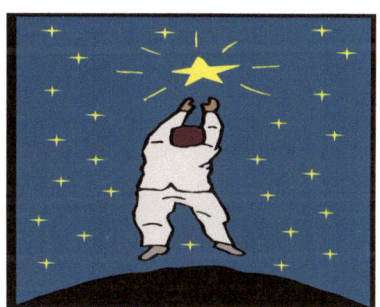

Wish 1

- Wish 1: Who do you want to make health care decisions for you if you cannot?

Think about the following:

❖ Do you want a healthcare proxy?

❖ If you want a healthcare proxy, Who do you wish to speak for you?

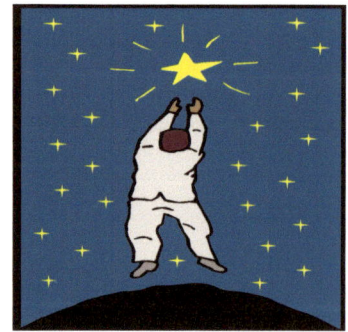

Wish 2

- Wish 2: What kind of medical care do you want or do not want?

Think about the following:

❖ Did you include what medical care you want or do not want in your living will?

❖ Were you specific about what medical treatments you want and do not want?

❖ Do you want a DNR order or a DNI?

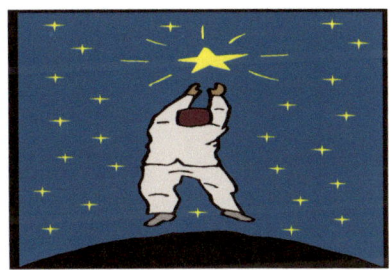

Wish 3

- Wish 3: How comfortable do I want to be?

Think about the following:

- ❖ What type of pain management do you want?

- ❖ What grooming and bathing instructions do you have?

- ❖ Do you want hospice care?

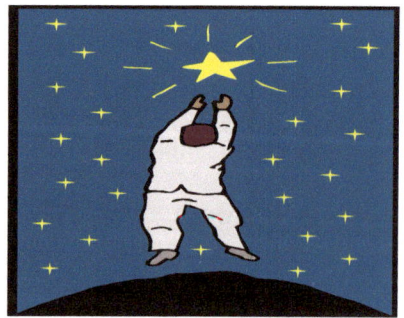

Wish 4

- Wish 4: How do you want people to treat you?

Think about the following:

❖ Do you want to be at home?

❖ Do you want someone praying beside you?

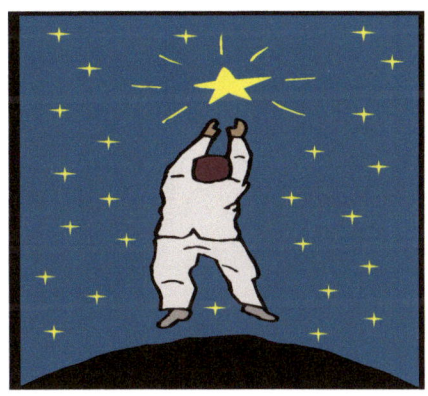

Wish 5

- Wish 5: What do you want your loved ones to know?

Think about the following:

❖ How do you want to be remembered?

❖ What final wishes do you want such as: burial, cremation and any special funeral or memorial plans?

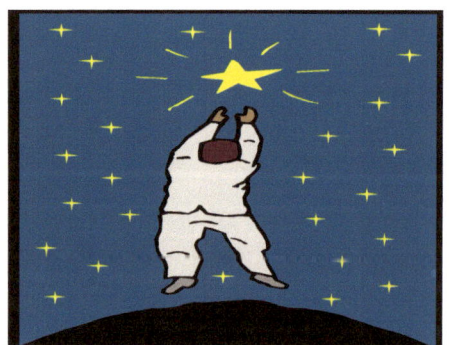

Common Question

- If I have a non-hospital DNR does this count in the hospital?

  ❖ Yes, in most states, a non-hospital DNR is treated the same as a hospital DNR until the attending doctor can examine you. It is not necessary for additional consents to be given. The doctor can order a hospital DNR.

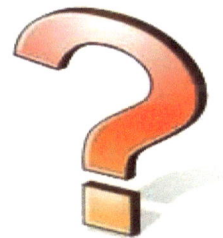

Common Question

- If I am transferred to another healthcare facility will my DNR be recognized?

  ❖ Yes, when transferred, the hospital will give EMS personnel the DNR order so that they in turn will give it to the healthcare facility you are transferred to.

What questions do you have?

It is important you discuss all questions with your nurse and doctor. Remember your nurse is your advocate and can help make sure all your healthcare wishes are followed.

Resources

Five wishes:

http://www.agingwithdignity.org/forms/5wishes.pdf

New York City Department of Health and Mental hygiene:

http://www.nyc.gov/html/doh/html/hca/advance-directives.shtml

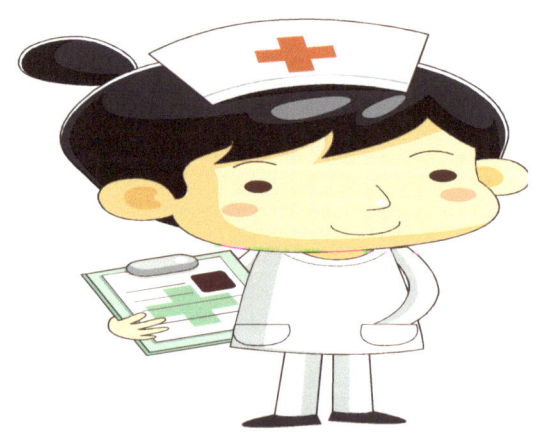

www.ingramcontent.com/pod-product-compliance
Lightning Source LLC
Chambersburg PA
CBHW041531280526
45792CB00004B/1457